21 Things to Create a Better Life

21 Things to Create a Better Life

Todd Bottorff

For my family.

Thank you.

Turner Publishing Company
200 4th Avenue North • Suite 950
Nashville, Tennessee 37219
(615) 255-2665

www.turnerpublishing.com

21 Things to Create a Better Life

Library of Congress Cataloging-in-Publication Data

Bottorff, Todd.
 21 things to create a better life / Todd Bottorff.
   p. cm.
 Includes bibliographical references.
 ISBN 978-1-59652-526-9
 1. Health. 2. Health behavior. 3. Courtesy. I. Title. II. Title: Twenty one things to create a better life.
 RA776.B669 2009
 613--dc22

                              2009000569

Printed in the United States of America

09 10 11 12 13 14 15 16—0 9 8 7 6 5 4 3 2 1

The passion of a heedless man grows like a creeper, and he runs from life to life, like a monkey seeking fruit in the forest.

Zen Saying

Don't give me the Zen, just tell me what to do.

Anonymous

Contents

Introduction:
The Problem and the Solution

Introduction

This book is about finding the easiest way to live a better life.

There are many books on this subject. What makes this book different is that it doesn't offer guiding principles or positive affirmations, it begins with simple, but powerful, actions. There are no platitudes here. For the saying that a 10,000-mile journey begins with a single step, these are the first steps. This book is for people who feel stressed or are looking for the easiest way to improve their lives within the constraints of real life.

The simplicity of the 21 things is deceptive. They appear small. But the reasoning behind them is powerful. Each item, alone, offers a positive benefit at minimal effort and cost. When added together, however, these 21 things provide a real path to monumental positive change.

The Problem

It can start in any area of your life. It could begin with high stress at work. It could begin with an injury. It could begin with having a child. Stress begins in one area of your life and flows into other areas—your sleep, your leisure, your relationships. Stress in one area of life affects another, and then another, until there is a downward pull on life generally. The negative flow has become a self-reinforcing cycle, undermining our human happiness.

The question is, How to reverse that cycle? Where to begin? Encouraging messages and uplifting affirmations are fine, but they don't solve the most difficult question: What is the first step to creating a better life?

The Solution

When we encounter stress, it would be wonderful to take a year off and move to the Australian outback or the Amalfi Coast or any other dreamy location, but realistically, not many of us have lives where time away is feasible. The challenge is that the forces that are causing stress are the same forces that lower our capacity to deal with stress, leading to the self-reinforcing negative cycle.

So where can you get a foothold when you have little time to dedicate to solving the problem? The answer is in activities that require minimal time and effort but have the greatest positive effect. The 21 Things are low-hassle, high-impact items that anyone can integrate into life. They cross a broad range of areas—wellness, relationships, financial health, and psychology. The 21 Things are arranged sequentially to coincide roughly with the routine of a typical day.

So the solution has two parts: the 21 things are

well selected and they are actionable. This combination provides a clear path to maximizing the benefits while minimizing the effort required.

Begin taking the first step to a better life with the simple plan that follows.

A Simple Plan

This plan moves your life from A to B. "A" is where you are now. "B" is a healthier, happier life. And the "to" is doing the 21 Things.

To break it down, the plan here is as follows:

1. Write down descriptions of various areas of your life as it is now (beginning on page 2).
2. Read the 21 Things.
3. Go to the final section of the book—21 Things for 21 Days—and check off the things as you do them for 21 days.
4. Write down descriptions of various areas of your life after the 21 days have passed (see page 118).

Your Life Now

On the next few pages, write descriptions of various aspects of your life. (Or if you prefer, just think about each of these and move on directly to the 21 Things.)

How would you describe the following areas of your life now?

Health and wellness

Date_____

Career or work

Date_____

Leisure activities

Date_____

Overall level of stress

Date_____

The 21 Things

– 1 –

Start the day with a glass of water

− 1 −

Start the day with a glass of water

A survey by the leading firm Yankelovich Partners for the Nutrition Information Center at the New York Hospital found that up to 75 percent of Americans are chronically dehydrated. As approximately 60 percent of our body weight is water and all of our systems are critically dependent on it, it only makes sense that we start the day with what we need most.

Morning is also the time of day when most people are naturally dehydrated because most will not have consumed any water for seven or more hours. It is at this point that we are at high risk of confusing hunger with thirst. A glass of water can prevent this confusion and adds zero calories to the diet. So satisfy the zero-calorie need first.

Starting the day with water is also an opportunity to luxuriate in small things. Try a variety of sources or no-calorie flavors of water served in various containers at different temperatures. Find the one you like best or vary them if that's your thing. A personal favorite is use of a filtered pitcher (such as a PUR pitcher) kept in the refrigerator, with service in a Tervis tumbler. There is something very satisfying about pure, cold water. Filtered pitchers also hold the advantage of being inexpensive compared with bottled water and minimizing the amount of plastic and its impact on the environment.

~ 2 ~

Eat breakfast like a king,
lunch like a prince,
and dinner like a pauper

Eat breakfast like a king, lunch like a prince, and dinner like a pauper

How many people rush into the day with a cup (or three) of coffee and a danish or doughnut, followed by a fast food lunch on the go, and take-out for dinner? This model seems to be standard fare in our high-stress world.

"Eat breakfast like a king" is an old saying, but it has been proven in medical studies to be valuable in achieving healthy living. As recently as June 2008, Dr. Daniela Jakubowicz, a clinical professor at Virginia Commonwealth University, presented the results of a study which concluded that a diet with a big breakfast resulted in five times the weight loss of one with a lower-calorie breakfast. Over eight months, an average of 40 pounds were shed by people enjoying a big breakfast versus 9 pounds by those with a light breakfast.

The challenge is how to make time to have a big breakfast. Most people are rushed in the mornings and don't find time for breakfast, or it consists of a stop at a drive-thru. One good option is microwaving an egg-white omelet with two pieces of toast, which can be done in the time it takes to drive through McDonalds. Other ideas are scheduling business breakfast meetings or finding a coffee shop located along the route to work.

The key is to set a starting day and choose to make it happen, then identify sources of food in advance consistent with your plan. There are two significant mistakes that people make. Either they don't eat or they make poor eating choices based on expediency. Don't just "grab something." If you choose to cook, decide what you are going to have and get the things you need in advance. If you are going to eat out, scout around in advance for a restaurant or coffee shop that meets your needs.

Having a big breakfast will curb the desire to snack or overeat at lunch and at dinner. The big breakfast may also enable you to incorporate time for a walk or leisure reading during lunch.

For lunch and dinner, set yourself up for success by identifying good choices for meals before you actually have to make the decision. By making good choices when you aren't hungry and in a rush, you lower the risk that lack of time will drive bad choices.

— 3 —

Turn off the radio in your car from time to time

Turn off the radio in your car from time to time

Nearly everyone has some form of audio going on in the car while driving. "An Exploratory Survey of In-Vehicle Music Listening" by Nicola Dibben and Victoria J. Williamson, published by Sage Journals in the United Kingdom in 2007, found that as many as 93 percent of drivers listen to some form of music or sound while driving.

Although music, radio programs, and conversation can be welcome distractions, the silence of the moment has value as well. Too often, audio becomes a habit. By turning off the radio from time to time, you remove the distraction and allow yourself to be more present with your own thoughts.

By removing the distraction you are also taking back control of your mental agenda. When you take back that space, you determine the programming. You can reflect on past events of the day, be present in the moment, or consider the future.

Try the peace and tranquillity of silence the next time you are in the car. Turn off the radio or mute the cell phone and enjoy the serenity of being alone with your thoughts.

— 4 —

Drink tea

– 4 –

Drink tea

The health benefits of drinking tea are significant and studies backing up its benign effects are numerous. Over thousands of years, tea has been proven to be beneficial to human health. The list of benefits includes quenching thirst, aiding digestion, preventing disease, strengthening bones, increasing mental focus while making you calm—and all at no calories.

Drinking tea is also another opportunity to luxuriate in the simplest of things. You can experiment with hot or cold tea; black, green, or red tea; you can go with loose tea, powdered tea, or tea bags. You can take a pragmatic approach with a travel mug or add ceremony with Asian tea sets. Whatever you choose, drinking tea is a good habit to have (with the caveat that heavily sugared tea is not among the healthy choices).

Consider this: If you currently grab a latte on the way to work, you are consuming 220 calories. That totals roughly 50,000 calories a year or the equivalent of 14 pounds of fat. Tea offers zero calories and no fat.

A personal favorite is Japanese green tea, and in particular, powdered Sencha from Den's Tea (find them online at www.denstea.com). They offer a starter sampler for trying a variety of teas at a very reasonable cost. So grab a mug and start drinking tea.

— 5 —

Get your news from a written format

Get your news from a written format

Everyone has heard the news mantra, "If it bleeds, it leads." Is this the guiding principle that you want controlling the information you receive about the world?

The revenue of television, radio, and Internet video is based solely on holding your attention. The things that most capture human attention are confrontational, shocking, dangerous, tragic, and terrifying. And the amount of broadcast time spent on any news story has been cut severely, limiting its ability to communicate any depth of thought about complex issues. Generating revenue by creating an emotional experience has eclipsed the journalistic ideal.

Try choosing a written format to get your news,

either on paper or electronic. Reading the news requires more concentration, which yields better retention and sharpens the ability to weigh the evidence and sift fact from fiction. It will give you greater control, provide better depth of coverage, reduce the number of shock images, and better represent the real issues that affect us.

The result is a more emotionally and intellectually mature understanding of the world. So choose a newspaper, journal, or Web site that offers objective, in-depth coverage of the issues and read when you would ordinarily watch the news.

– 6 –

Don't pick the closest parking space

– 6 –

Don't pick the closest parking space

Given that the average person parks somewhere twice daily, by not picking the closest parking space, that person could walk an additional 35 miles annually. Depending on weight and pace that would be something like lopping off 3,500 calories a year or the equivalent of one pound of fat. A simple thing, but enough to eliminate the average midlife weight gain of half a pound a year.

In addition, it eliminates the performance stress caused by the self-imposed requirement of having to select the single closest space. Barry Schwartz describes this phenomenon in his thoughtful book *The Paradox of Choice.* By having so many options and forcing ourselves to choose the "best" one, we impose a performance anxiety on ourselves. Ironic, isn't it, that we stress over making a choice where getting the best outcome is doing us harm?

— 7 —

Agree when you can, look for a joint solution when you can't

Agree when you can, look for a joint solution when you can't

When did there arise such a premium on confrontation?

It doesn't take a lot of analysis to determine that much of our national dialogue is based on conflict. We seem to be focused on what divides us rather than on the things we share. Much of this disagreement is unnecessary and counterproductive. But agreement and compromise do not make for good drama and therefore are downplayed by the media.

In this environment it is all the more important to make sure that we don't apply a confrontational model to our real lives. When we interact with others and there seems to be disagreement, if we begin with the things that divide us, the problem-solving approach can degenerate into a straight negotiation or argument where each party applies power to achieve the objective. Even if one party "wins," a negative sentiment created by the argument survives.

In order to build relationships with the capacity and patience for working through disagreements in a positive way, the first step is to affirm the things that both parties agree on. Once these elements have been identified, isolate the issue causing disagreement while affirming that the goal is to find a solution that works for both sides. Then suggest a compromise and solicit possible solutions from the other party.

This approach works in every situation from serving in Congress to picking up the dry cleaning. Even when no compromise is available, going through these steps of human interaction shows mutual respect. By applying this approach, you will make your human interaction as positive as it can be, which is a good foundation for building good relationships.

When you feel the urge to engage in conflict, apply this approach: affirm what you can agree on, suggest a compromise in the form of a question, and ask for alternatives in return. When applied to negotiation, this model helps eliminate conflict by curbing negative emotions, thereby lowering stress.

– 8 –

Take a moment to be where you are

− 8 −

Take a moment to be where you are

A few weeks ago I was at lunch with a friend. At the table nearest us sat two young women. Each was texting away and neither was interacting with the other.

If you look at the daily amount of time people spend engaging with technology—the Internet, the Blackberry, cell phones, iPhones, MP3 players—designed to allow you to connect with someplace else, you may be shocked.

Although these technologies allow greater connectedness, paradoxically the connectedness they make possible disconnects our attention from our present reality. And there is no technological substitute for reality.

Managing when to be engaged in the present and when to utilize technological tools to connect to someplace else is an important skill. So the next time you are looking at checking your email on a mobile device or texting away, ask yourself, Is this more important than giving full attention to the present reality, whether that includes interacting with others or just being alone with the surrounding environment?

— 9 —

Say "please," "thank you," and "you're welcome"

Say "please," "thank you," and "you're welcome"

It seems so obvious. We should all be more polite. But a look at the sociology behind the rationale for polite speech may be more motivating.

George Homans, one of the most influential sociologists of the twentieth century, completed numerous studies on human interaction. Using a simplified version of his framework, the rationale goes like this: positive interaction contributes to positive sentiment, and positive sentiments contribute to positive relationships. In turn, positive relationships contribute immensely to human happiness.

There is no easier way to contribute to positive sentiment between yourself and others than simple, sincere, polite speech. It's free. There is no downside to using it. The amount of effort is negligible and the benefits can be substantial.

So, take a day, any day, and consider how many times you say "please," "thank you," and "you're welcome" versus the number of times you ask someone for something, you receive something from someone, or someone says "thank you" to you. You may find you have many opportunities to add these simple words benefiting yourself and others.

~ 10 ~

Wash your hands

Wash your hands

It seems fundamental, but the reality is somewhat disturbing.

In a Harris Interactive survey prepared for the American Society for Microbiology, observers recorded the percentage of adults who washed their hands in six public restrooms across the country. The restrooms were equipped with soap and towels, so real-world percentages could be even smaller when taking into account restrooms that are out of soap and towels. In the survey, 92 percent of people said they wash their hands, but only 83 percent actually did. Women washed more at 90 percent, and only 75 percent of the men washed their hands. These figures do not include the number of people who do not wash their hands after sneezing, coughing, and other necessities.

The number of illnesses and diseases that can be prevented by this simple activity cannot be accurately quantified because to date no study has linked the absence of hand washing to other human interaction such as shaking hands, or to turning a doorknob or using a shopping cart. But washing hands has been proven to prevent transfer of the common cold virus, influenza, and foodborne pathogens. Infectious disease is the largest cause of death globally and third in the U.S.

The Centers for Disease Control and Prevention recommends that you wash with warm water and soap for 15 to 20 seconds after using the restroom, before handling food, after coughing or sneezing, after caring for the sick, and after touching animals. A complete guideline is available at cleanhandscoalition.org.

So, if you want to be healthy, wash your hands.

– 11 –

Put your household budget on paper (and get into the black)

─ 11 ─

Put your household budget on paper (and get into the black)

This is a big one. The overall process of reaching financial health is much greater than the scope of this book, but the simple thing that you can do is to compile your data and put your household budget on paper.

A survey by the legal Web site findlaw.com found that 30 percent of Americans have no household budget. To some the word "budget" carries a negative connotation. It shouldn't. The exercise of committing things to paper is the first step to being aware, and awareness is the first step to making good financial decisions that lead to fiscal health. All you need is paper, a pen, a calculator, and a few documents.

The easy way to do this:

1. Get a copy of the most recent paycheck (or an average one if your income varies) from all earners in your household (don't include any money realized from borrowing or selling assets).

2. Write down your average monthly pre-tax income (the amount before taxes are deducted).

3. Subtract income taxes you pay (withholding, payroll, etc.). You now have your after-tax income ("take-home pay").

4. Collect your bills for the preceding few months—mortgage or rent, home maintenance, electricity, water, natural gas, phone, TV, grocery, credit card bills, auto loan or lease, gasoline, any other loans, and so forth.

5. Get a copy of your bank statement and check all subtractions from your account to make sure all expenses are covered.

6. Rank them from largest to smallest.

7. Add them up to get your total expenses.

Subtract the total expenses from the after-tax income. There are many complexities to making suggestions about how to manage all these items, but the key thing is, if the number you have left is negative (in the "red"), you have taken the first step to financial health by recognizing there is a problem. Now you can get some assistance and start making some changes. A good resource to consider is Dave Ramsey's book *The Total Money Makeover.*

If the number is positive (in the "black"), congratulations! You have the flexibility to start building wealth.

~ 12 ~

Only use debt to buy appreciating assets

━ 12 ━

Only use debt to buy appreciating assets

A look at the increase in household debt among Americans paints a worrisome picture. In 1983, household debt was 40 percent of GDP, our country's gross economic output. Today household debt is at 100 percent of GDP. So we have a lot more debt relative to the size of our economy than we did 25 years ago. The key question is, What is that debt being used to buy?

If the debt is buying assets whose values grow more than the debt costs over the long-term, then our net worth is going up. If it is buying Xboxes, lattes, automobiles, and trips to the Bahamas, then we are on our way to becoming a very poor country. The facts are, it is a mixture of both, but far too many of us are using debt for a purpose that will make us poorer. And if enough people use debt unwisely, those who use it wisely will suffer also.

Learning to make wise buying choices is a process that could take a long time, but the key is to begin making daily decisions that move you the right direction toward that goal.

If you are going to take on debt, use it to buy appreciating assets only. The additional caveat is that you have to have enough equity (cash that you don't need for living expenses) to ride out the ups and downs in value. But what is an appreciating asset?

An appreciating asset is something that generally goes up in value. The term "generally" is used because nearly all assets have periods where their values decline. Assets that fall into this group are stocks and bonds, real estate, collectibles, and so forth. It is important to recognize that not all the things that fall into these categories will appreciate. Some stocks will go down and never rise again, and most assets will have periods where their values drop. You need enough diversification (in stocks, for example) to increase the likelihood that your asset will rise in value. You also need to have enough of a cushion to weather the declines. The way to figure out how much of a cushion you need is to look at how much the value can drop at any one time, then put enough equity in at the start so that if it does drop, the value of the asset minus the debt is always a positive number and your after-tax income can cover the cost of holding it—which is the interest, plus any principal due, plus taxes and maintenance.

What isn't an appreciating asset? This group includes depreciating assets or expenses. Here "depreciating" means assets with a market value that generally goes only down (not assets where the accounting term "depreciation" applies). Things like cars and new furniture are depreciating assets. Things like travel, clothes, food, and toys are expenses, meaning their value very quickly goes to zero or close to it.

The next time you plan to borrow money, ask yourself these questions: Am I using this money to buy an appreciating asset and do I have enough of an equity cushion? If the answer to either is "no," walk away and go treat yourself to an ice cream cone instead.

– 13 –

Don't eat in the two hours before bed

– 13 –

Don't eat in the two hours before bed

Sleep studies indicate that eating just before going to bed undermines the ability to get a good night's sleep. Reaching deep sleep is a critical part of the body's ability to heal itself, both mentally and physically. You should also avoid alcohol and caffeine during these hours to increase your chances of getting a good night's sleep.

Although this idea is well known, the question is, How do you make it happen? One suggestion is to "close the kitchen" during this time. Closing it means cleaning up, putting everything away, and turning out the lights. This action creates a mental break between where and when you eat and when you don't. Also avoid watching TV commercials during this time.

Make it easier on yourself by eliminating the hundreds of images of pizza, tacos, chicken, and burgers typically aired in the evening hours. You can either avoid TV altogether, watch something that doesn't run commercials, or fast-forward through them with a digital video recorder.

— 14 —

Walk a little bit after dinner

～ 14 ～

Walk a little bit after dinner

How many of us habitually eat dinner and then move straight to the couch, if we aren't already there?

I learned of the impact of this ritual from a friend. His wife was pregnant with their first child. She was diagnosed with borderline gestational diabetes. The recommendation was to get a glucose meter and to make changes in diet and exercise. After eating, her blood sugar would spike. To manage it she began taking a short walk, to the end of the block and back for example. This walk lowered the spike dramatically. The couple told me how amazed they were to learn how much the glucose numbers improved.

Creating the ritual of a short walk after dinner carries remarkable benefits for your health and your mind and breaks the habit of dinner-to-couch. So try walking a bit after dinner. The impact will improve your physical and mental health, and state of mind, and help to break sedentary habits.

— 15 —

Hug your spouse or significant other for at least a minute every day

Hug your spouse or significant other for at least a minute every day

How many days a week do you hug your spouse or significant other?

The schedule, the rush, the demands on our time, they all work against this simple thing, but medical research is now realizing a greater understanding of how important this show of affection is to our health and our relationships.

Kathleen Light at the University of North Carolina Chapel Hill found that warm contact aided in the production of the hormone oxytocin, which appeared to have a positive effect in the lowering of stress and blood pressure. In her study, couples committed to a "brief episode of warm contact," and embrace, had higher levels of oxytocin.

So take a minute to hug your spouse or significant other. It is the best, free, 100 percent healthy drug you can find.

~ 16 ~

Stretch

— 16 —

Stretch

The effects of stretching extend beyond increased flexibility—stretching increases blood flow, reduces the risk of injury, enhances muscle relaxation, and much more. In a few minutes a person of almost any fitness level can utilize simple stretches to improve physical and mental health.

The image of suiting up and taking an hour to visit the gym, the park, or the yoga studio, while nice, is not necessary to achieving measurable health benefits. Try integrating a few minutes of stretching at various times throughout the day to maintain energy at work or at home.

Some helpful resources are Bob Anderson's book, simply titled *Stretching,* and the book *Stretching*

Anatomy by Arnold Nelson. Many of the exercises in these books can be performed during your normal day: at your desk, before bed, even in the elevator (it might be best if you are alone for that one).

— 17 —

Read before bed

– 17 –

Read before bed

A survey conducted by mattress manufacturer Serta on the sleeping habits of Americans found that three-quarters of Americans reported that watching TV is their primary pre-bedtime ritual.

University of Maryland researchers John Robinson and Steve Martin collected social data and media usage from more than 45,000 people. Their survey found that people who watched more television reported being less happy. Although the survey could not assert underlying causes, is it any wonder that with the great number of disturbing images on television, large numbers of people cannot get a good night's sleep? According to the National Commission on Sleep Disorders, 60 to 70 million Americans have difficulty sleeping.

There are more than four million books in print. They exist on nearly every subject, fiction and nonfiction. Reading quiets the mind and makes you a more knowledgeable, interesting person.

By turning off the TV and picking up the book, you increase your chances of a good night's sleep. You gain all the benefits of reading as well as the benefits of a restful night.

Pick anything you are interested in. Get a book on the subject. Lay the book on your bedside table and read a little bit before bed. You'll sleep better, you'll know more, and good things will follow.

~ 18 ~

Floss

– 18 –

Floss

Your dentist tells you this every time you visit about how flossing will prevent tooth decay and periodontal disease, but what you may not know is that now more evidence is emerging that it may help to prevent heart disease, America's number-one cause of death as reported by the Centers for Disease Control and Prevention.

The *Journal of Periodontology* reported in two studies that the same bacteria that appear in plaque around your teeth also contribute to a greater risk of heart attack. These bacteria can be removed by flossing. So flossing serves as a filter, removing dangerous bacteria and thereby reducing the chance of heart attack.

For the two minutes it takes to floss your teeth, you can improve your relationships, reduce your dental bills, and prolong your life.

— 19 —

Take five deep breaths

~ 19 ~

Take five deep breaths

Almost anyone can find the time to take five deep breaths. The effects can be significantly positive. From lower blood pressure to reduced stress, breathing is a free, zero-calorie, highly portable activity.

In his book *Free Your Breath, Free Your Life,* Dennis Lewis provides a comprehensive guide to deep breathing and its benefits. There is a lot more to breathing deeply than just taking five deep breaths, but for the vast majority of people who never think about their breathing, simply taking five is a start.

— 20 —

Count your blessings

– 20 –

Count your blessings

In this performance-oriented world, there is a tendency to focus on the small percentage of things that need improvement. How else can we improve but by examining what is wrong? The trouble arises when such thinking leads us to put a lower valuation on the quality of our lives.

It is easy to fall into the trap of allowing anxiety to drive your thinking, especially when your head hits the pillow. Some people describe this pitfall as allowing the mind to run through a litany of worries, bouncing from one to the next, and never actually applying any productive thought to them.

In order to break this habit, actively think about the large percentage of things that you have that are ideal or wonderful. If you are religious you can do this in prayer. The glass is typically much more than half full if you allow yourself to see it that way.

~ 21 ~

When your head hits the pillow, smile

— 21 —

When your head hits the pillow, smile

Although it sounds somewhat silly, there is medical evidence in support of the psychological benefits of smiling.

In his book *Emotions Revealed,* Paul Ekman provides a fascinating discussion about reading people's emotions based on their expressions. In the book he asserts that when subjects experimented by imitating certain expressions, they would begin to actually feel the emotions they imitated. The theory is that the human body generates the chemicals that make you feel the emotions when your muscles exhibit those emotions.

What's more, *The British Medical Journal* completed a study in December 2008 asserting that happiness is contagious. The study found that people who interact with others who are happy increase their own chances of being happy.

So, if you want to feel happier, smile.

21 Things for 21 Days

There are various theories on how long it takes to develop a habit, either positive or negative. To simplify them, the three largest schools of thought are that it takes either 21 days, 6 weeks, or 90 days depending on how you look at it.

Each theory has its merits and the differences can be reconciled by how effective or long-lasting the "habit" tends to be. If an activity is repeated for 21 days, a real change in behavior is likely, but the risk is greater of its not enduring. At 6 weeks, a habit has a much greater chance of enduring, but the associated physiological changes in our brains and our bodies remain incomplete. At 90 days, there are measurable physiological changes that reset the behavior as the norm, which requires further changes in order to be modified. This is why many programs dedicated to changing life's habits use the 90-day model.

Regardless of which definition seems most compelling to you, all change is about one day—today—and the actions you take in the present.

The template on the following pages is a tool for recording the 21 Things the first 21 days you repeat them. The act of checking off the 21 Things as you do them itself can become a positive habit. It creates personal accountability and marks progress. So pick your day and get started. At the end of the 21 days, complete the personal inventory questionnaire. You may copy the blank questionnaire (beginning on page 118) to use if you would like to continue the 21 Things through 6 weeks or 90 days or beyond.

Best wishes and congratulations on the courage to do the first thing!

Day _____

- ☐ Start the day with a glass of water
- ☐ Eat breakfast like a king, lunch like a prince, and dinner like a pauper
- ☐ Turn off the radio in your car from time to time
- ☐ Drink tea
- ☐ Get your news from a written format
- ☐ Don't pick the closest parking space
- ☐ Agree when you can, look for a joint solution when you can't
- ☐ Take a moment to be where you are
- ☐ Say "please," "thank you," and "you're welcome"
- ☐ Wash your hands
- ☐ Put your household budget on paper (and get into the black)
- ☐ Only use debt to buy appreciating assets
- ☐ Don't eat in the two hours before bed
- ☐ Walk a little bit after dinner
- ☐ Hug your spouse or significant other for at least a minute every day
- ☐ Stretch
- ☐ Read before bed
- ☐ Floss
- ☐ Take five deep breaths
- ☐ Count your blessings
- ☐ When your head hits the pillow, smile

Day _____

- ☐ Start the day with a glass of water
- ☐ Eat breakfast like a king, lunch like a prince, and dinner like a pauper
- ☐ Turn off the radio in your car from time to time
- ☐ Drink tea
- ☐ Get your news from a written format
- ☐ Don't pick the closest parking space
- ☐ Agree when you can, look for a joint solution when you can't
- ☐ Take a moment to be where you are
- ☐ Say "please," "thank you," and "you're welcome"
- ☐ Wash your hands
- ☐ Put your household budget on paper (and get into the black)
- ☐ Only use debt to buy appreciating assets
- ☐ Don't eat in the two hours before bed
- ☐ Walk a little bit after dinner
- ☐ Hug your spouse or significant other for at least a minute every day
- ☐ Stretch
- ☐ Read before bed
- ☐ Floss
- ☐ Take five deep breaths
- ☐ Count your blessings
- ☐ When your head hits the pillow, smile

Day _____

- ☐ Start the day with a glass of water
- ☐ Eat breakfast like a king, lunch like a prince, and dinner like a pauper
- ☐ Turn off the radio in your car from time to time
- ☐ Drink tea
- ☐ Get your news from a written format
- ☐ Don't pick the closest parking space
- ☐ Agree when you can, look for a joint solution when you can't
- ☐ Take a moment to be where you are
- ☐ Say "please," "thank you," and "you're welcome"
- ☐ Wash your hands
- ☐ Put your household budget on paper (and get into the black)
- ☐ Only use debt to buy appreciating assets
- ☐ Don't eat in the two hours before bed
- ☐ Walk a little bit after dinner
- ☐ Hug your spouse or significant other for at least a minute every day
- ☐ Stretch
- ☐ Read before bed
- ☐ Floss
- ☐ Take five deep breaths
- ☐ Count your blessings
- ☐ When your head hits the pillow, smile

Day _____

- ☐ Start the day with a glass of water
- ☐ Eat breakfast like a king, lunch like a prince, and dinner like a pauper
- ☐ Turn off the radio in your car from time to time
- ☐ Drink tea
- ☐ Get your news from a written format
- ☐ Don't pick the closest parking space
- ☐ Agree when you can, look for a joint solution when you can't
- ☐ Take a moment to be where you are
- ☐ Say "please," "thank you," and "you're welcome"
- ☐ Wash your hands
- ☐ Put your household budget on paper (and get into the black)
- ☐ Only use debt to buy appreciating assets
- ☐ Don't eat in the two hours before bed
- ☐ Walk a little bit after dinner
- ☐ Hug your spouse or significant other for at least a minute every day
- ☐ Stretch
- ☐ Read before bed
- ☐ Floss
- ☐ Take five deep breaths
- ☐ Count your blessings
- ☐ When your head hits the pillow, smile

Day _____

- ☐ Start the day with a glass of water
- ☐ Eat breakfast like a king, lunch like a prince, and dinner like a pauper
- ☐ Turn off the radio in your car from time to time
- ☐ Drink tea
- ☐ Get your news from a written format
- ☐ Don't pick the closest parking space
- ☐ Agree when you can, look for a joint solution when you can't
- ☐ Take a moment to be where you are
- ☐ Say "please," "thank you," and "you're welcome"
- ☐ Wash your hands
- ☐ Put your household budget on paper (and get into the black)
- ☐ Only use debt to buy appreciating assets
- ☐ Don't eat in the two hours before bed
- ☐ Walk a little bit after dinner
- ☐ Hug your spouse or significant other for at least a minute every day
- ☐ Stretch
- ☐ Read before bed
- ☐ Floss
- ☐ Take five deep breaths
- ☐ Count your blessings
- ☐ When your head hits the pillow, smile

Day _____

- [ ] Start the day with a glass of water
- [ ] Eat breakfast like a king, lunch like a prince, and dinner like a pauper
- [ ] Turn off the radio in your car from time to time
- [ ] Drink tea
- [ ] Get your news from a written format
- [ ] Don't pick the closest parking space
- [ ] Agree when you can, look for a joint solution when you can't
- [ ] Take a moment to be where you are
- [ ] Say "please," "thank you," and "you're welcome"
- [ ] Wash your hands
- [ ] Put your household budget on paper (and get into the black)
- [ ] Only use debt to buy appreciating assets
- [ ] Don't eat in the two hours before bed
- [ ] Walk a little bit after dinner
- [ ] Hug your spouse or significant other for at least a minute every day
- [ ] Stretch
- [ ] Read before bed
- [ ] Floss
- [ ] Take five deep breaths
- [ ] Count your blessings
- [ ] When your head hits the pillow, smile

Day _____

- ☐ Start the day with a glass of water
- ☐ Eat breakfast like a king, lunch like a prince, and dinner like a pauper
- ☐ Turn off the radio in your car from time to time
- ☐ Drink tea
- ☐ Get your news from a written format
- ☐ Don't pick the closest parking space
- ☐ Agree when you can, look for a joint solution when you can't
- ☐ Take a moment to be where you are
- ☐ Say "please," "thank you," and "you're welcome"
- ☐ Wash your hands
- ☐ Put your household budget on paper (and get into the black)
- ☐ Only use debt to buy appreciating assets
- ☐ Don't eat in the two hours before bed
- ☐ Walk a little bit after dinner
- ☐ Hug your spouse or significant other for at least a minute every day
- ☐ Stretch
- ☐ Read before bed
- ☐ Floss
- ☐ Take five deep breaths
- ☐ Count your blessings
- ☐ When your head hits the pillow, smile

Day _____

- [ ] Start the day with a glass of water
- [ ] Eat breakfast like a king, lunch like a prince, and dinner like a pauper
- [ ] Turn off the radio in your car from time to time
- [ ] Drink tea
- [ ] Get your news from a written format
- [ ] Don't pick the closest parking space
- [ ] Agree when you can, look for a joint solution when you can't
- [ ] Take a moment to be where you are
- [ ] Say "please," "thank you," and "you're welcome"
- [ ] Wash your hands
- [ ] Put your household budget on paper (and get into the black)
- [ ] Only use debt to buy appreciating assets
- [ ] Don't eat in the two hours before bed
- [ ] Walk a little bit after dinner
- [ ] Hug your spouse or significant other for at least a minute every day
- [ ] Stretch
- [ ] Read before bed
- [ ] Floss
- [ ] Take five deep breaths
- [ ] Count your blessings
- [ ] When your head hits the pillow, smile

Day _____

- ☐ Start the day with a glass of water
- ☐ Eat breakfast like a king, lunch like a prince, and dinner like a pauper
- ☐ Turn off the radio in your car from time to time
- ☐ Drink tea
- ☐ Get your news from a written format
- ☐ Don't pick the closest parking space
- ☐ Agree when you can, look for a joint solution when you can't
- ☐ Take a moment to be where you are
- ☐ Say "please," "thank you," and "you're welcome"
- ☐ Wash your hands
- ☐ Put your household budget on paper (and get into the black)
- ☐ Only use debt to buy appreciating assets
- ☐ Don't eat in the two hours before bed
- ☐ Walk a little bit after dinner
- ☐ Hug your spouse or significant other for at least a minute every day
- ☐ Stretch
- ☐ Read before bed
- ☐ Floss
- ☐ Take five deep breaths
- ☐ Count your blessings
- ☐ When your head hits the pillow, smile

Day _____

- [ ] Start the day with a glass of water
- [ ] Eat breakfast like a king, lunch like a prince, and dinner like a pauper
- [ ] Turn off the radio in your car from time to time
- [ ] Drink tea
- [ ] Get your news from a written format
- [ ] Don't pick the closest parking space
- [ ] Agree when you can, look for a joint solution when you can't
- [ ] Take a moment to be where you are
- [ ] Say "please," "thank you," and "you're welcome"
- [ ] Wash your hands
- [ ] Put your household budget on paper (and get into the black)
- [ ] Only use debt to buy appreciating assets
- [ ] Don't eat in the two hours before bed
- [ ] Walk a little bit after dinner
- [ ] Hug your spouse or significant other for at least a minute every day
- [ ] Stretch
- [ ] Read before bed
- [ ] Floss
- [ ] Take five deep breaths
- [ ] Count your blessings
- [ ] When your head hits the pillow, smile

Day _____

- ☐ Start the day with a glass of water
- ☐ Eat breakfast like a king, lunch like a prince, and dinner like a pauper
- ☐ Turn off the radio in your car from time to time
- ☐ Drink tea
- ☐ Get your news from a written format
- ☐ Don't pick the closest parking space
- ☐ Agree when you can, look for a joint solution when you can't
- ☐ Take a moment to be where you are
- ☐ Say "please," "thank you," and "you're welcome"
- ☐ Wash your hands
- ☐ Put your household budget on paper (and get into the black)
- ☐ Only use debt to buy appreciating assets
- ☐ Don't eat in the two hours before bed
- ☐ Walk a little bit after dinner
- ☐ Hug your spouse or significant other for at least a minute every day
- ☐ Stretch
- ☐ Read before bed
- ☐ Floss
- ☐ Take five deep breaths
- ☐ Count your blessings
- ☐ When your head hits the pillow, smile

Day _____

- ☐ Start the day with a glass of water
- ☐ Eat breakfast like a king, lunch like a prince, and dinner like a pauper
- ☐ Turn off the radio in your car from time to time
- ☐ Drink tea
- ☐ Get your news from a written format
- ☐ Don't pick the closest parking space
- ☐ Agree when you can, look for a joint solution when you can't
- ☐ Take a moment to be where you are
- ☐ Say "please," "thank you," and "you're welcome"
- ☐ Wash your hands
- ☐ Put your household budget on paper (and get into the black)
- ☐ Only use debt to buy appreciating assets
- ☐ Don't eat in the two hours before bed
- ☐ Walk a little bit after dinner
- ☐ Hug your spouse or significant other for at least a minute every day
- ☐ Stretch
- ☐ Read before bed
- ☐ Floss
- ☐ Take five deep breaths
- ☐ Count your blessings
- ☐ When your head hits the pillow, smile

Day _____

- ☐ Start the day with a glass of water
- ☐ Eat breakfast like a king, lunch like a prince, and dinner like a pauper
- ☐ Turn off the radio in your car from time to time
- ☐ Drink tea
- ☐ Get your news from a written format
- ☐ Don't pick the closest parking space
- ☐ Agree when you can, look for a joint solution when you can't
- ☐ Take a moment to be where you are
- ☐ Say "please," "thank you," and "you're welcome"
- ☐ Wash your hands
- ☐ Put your household budget on paper (and get into the black)
- ☐ Only use debt to buy appreciating assets
- ☐ Don't eat in the two hours before bed
- ☐ Walk a little bit after dinner
- ☐ Hug your spouse or significant other for at least a minute every day
- ☐ Stretch
- ☐ Read before bed
- ☐ Floss
- ☐ Take five deep breaths
- ☐ Count your blessings
- ☐ When your head hits the pillow, smile

Day _____

- [ ] Start the day with a glass of water
- [ ] Eat breakfast like a king, lunch like a prince, and dinner like a pauper
- [ ] Turn off the radio in your car from time to time
- [ ] Drink tea
- [ ] Get your news from a written format
- [ ] Don't pick the closest parking space
- [ ] Agree when you can, look for a joint solution when you can't
- [ ] Take a moment to be where you are
- [ ] Say "please," "thank you," and "you're welcome"
- [ ] Wash your hands
- [ ] Put your household budget on paper (and get into the black)
- [ ] Only use debt to buy appreciating assets
- [ ] Don't eat in the two hours before bed
- [ ] Walk a little bit after dinner
- [ ] Hug your spouse or significant other for at least a minute every day
- [ ] Stretch
- [ ] Read before bed
- [ ] Floss
- [ ] Take five deep breaths
- [ ] Count your blessings
- [ ] When your head hits the pillow, smile

Day _____

- ☐ Start the day with a glass of water
- ☐ Eat breakfast like a king, lunch like a prince, and dinner like a pauper
- ☐ Turn off the radio in your car from time to time
- ☐ Drink tea
- ☐ Get your news from a written format
- ☐ Don't pick the closest parking space
- ☐ Agree when you can, look for a joint solution when you can't
- ☐ Take a moment to be where you are
- ☐ Say "please," "thank you," and "you're welcome"
- ☐ Wash your hands
- ☐ Put your household budget on paper (and get into the black)
- ☐ Only use debt to buy appreciating assets
- ☐ Don't eat in the two hours before bed
- ☐ Walk a little bit after dinner
- ☐ Hug your spouse or significant other for at least a minute every day
- ☐ Stretch
- ☐ Read before bed
- ☐ Floss
- ☐ Take five deep breaths
- ☐ Count your blessings
- ☐ When your head hits the pillow, smile

Day _____

- ☐ Start the day with a glass of water
- ☐ Eat breakfast like a king, lunch like a prince, and dinner like a pauper
- ☐ Turn off the radio in your car from time to time
- ☐ Drink tea
- ☐ Get your news from a written format
- ☐ Don't pick the closest parking space
- ☐ Agree when you can, look for a joint solution when you can't
- ☐ Take a moment to be where you are
- ☐ Say "please," "thank you," and "you're welcome"
- ☐ Wash your hands
- ☐ Put your household budget on paper (and get into the black)
- ☐ Only use debt to buy appreciating assets
- ☐ Don't eat in the two hours before bed
- ☐ Walk a little bit after dinner
- ☐ Hug your spouse or significant other for at least a minute every day
- ☐ Stretch
- ☐ Read before bed
- ☐ Floss
- ☐ Take five deep breaths
- ☐ Count your blessings
- ☐ When your head hits the pillow, smile

Day _____

- ☐ Start the day with a glass of water
- ☐ Eat breakfast like a king, lunch like a prince, and dinner like a pauper
- ☐ Turn off the radio in your car from time to time
- ☐ Drink tea
- ☐ Get your news from a written format
- ☐ Don't pick the closest parking space
- ☐ Agree when you can, look for a joint solution when you can't
- ☐ Take a moment to be where you are
- ☐ Say "please," "thank you," and "you're welcome"
- ☐ Wash your hands
- ☐ Put your household budget on paper (and get into the black)
- ☐ Only use debt to buy appreciating assets
- ☐ Don't eat in the two hours before bed
- ☐ Walk a little bit after dinner
- ☐ Hug your spouse or significant other for at least a minute every day
- ☐ Stretch
- ☐ Read before bed
- ☐ Floss
- ☐ Take five deep breaths
- ☐ Count your blessings
- ☐ When your head hits the pillow, smile

Day _____

- [ ] Start the day with a glass of water
- [ ] Eat breakfast like a king, lunch like a prince, and dinner like a pauper
- [ ] Turn off the radio in your car from time to time
- [ ] Drink tea
- [ ] Get your news from a written format
- [ ] Don't pick the closest parking space
- [ ] Agree when you can, look for a joint solution when you can't
- [ ] Take a moment to be where you are
- [ ] Say "please," "thank you," and "you're welcome"
- [ ] Wash your hands
- [ ] Put your household budget on paper (and get into the black)
- [ ] Only use debt to buy appreciating assets
- [ ] Don't eat in the two hours before bed
- [ ] Walk a little bit after dinner
- [ ] Hug your spouse or significant other for at least a minute every day
- [ ] Stretch
- [ ] Read before bed
- [ ] Floss
- [ ] Take five deep breaths
- [ ] Count your blessings
- [ ] When your head hits the pillow, smile

Day _____

- ☐ Start the day with a glass of water
- ☐ Eat breakfast like a king, lunch like a prince, and dinner like a pauper
- ☐ Turn off the radio in your car from time to time
- ☐ Drink tea
- ☐ Get your news from a written format
- ☐ Don't pick the closest parking space
- ☐ Agree when you can, look for a joint solution when you can't
- ☐ Take a moment to be where you are
- ☐ Say "please," "thank you," and "you're welcome"
- ☐ Wash your hands
- ☐ Put your household budget on paper (and get into the black)
- ☐ Only use debt to buy appreciating assets
- ☐ Don't eat in the two hours before bed
- ☐ Walk a little bit after dinner
- ☐ Hug your spouse or significant other for at least a minute every day
- ☐ Stretch
- ☐ Read before bed
- ☐ Floss
- ☐ Take five deep breaths
- ☐ Count your blessings
- ☐ When your head hits the pillow, smile

Day _____

- ☐ Start the day with a glass of water
- ☐ Eat breakfast like a king, lunch like a prince, and dinner like a pauper
- ☐ Turn off the radio in your car from time to time
- ☐ Drink tea
- ☐ Get your news from a written format
- ☐ Don't pick the closest parking space
- ☐ Agree when you can, look for a joint solution when you can't
- ☐ Take a moment to be where you are
- ☐ Say "please," "thank you," and "you're welcome"
- ☐ Wash your hands
- ☐ Put your household budget on paper (and get into the black)
- ☐ Only use debt to buy appreciating assets
- ☐ Don't eat in the two hours before bed
- ☐ Walk a little bit after dinner
- ☐ Hug your spouse or significant other for at least a minute every day
- ☐ Stretch
- ☐ Read before bed
- ☐ Floss
- ☐ Take five deep breaths
- ☐ Count your blessings
- ☐ When your head hits the pillow, smile

Day _____

- ☐ Start the day with a glass of water
- ☐ Eat breakfast like a king, lunch like a prince, and dinner like a pauper
- ☐ Turn off the radio in your car from time to time
- ☐ Drink tea
- ☐ Get your news from a written format
- ☐ Don't pick the closest parking space
- ☐ Agree when you can, look for a joint solution when you can't
- ☐ Take a moment to be where you are
- ☐ Say "please," "thank you," and "you're welcome"
- ☐ Wash your hands
- ☐ Put your household budget on paper (and get into the black)
- ☐ Only use debt to buy appreciating assets
- ☐ Don't eat in the two hours before bed
- ☐ Walk a little bit after dinner
- ☐ Hug your spouse or significant other for at least a minute every day
- ☐ Stretch
- ☐ Read before bed
- ☐ Floss
- ☐ Take five deep breaths
- ☐ Count your blessings
- ☐ When your head hits the pillow, smile

Your Life at the End
of the 21 Days

How would you describe the following areas of your life now?

On the next few pages, write descriptions of various aspects of your life.

Health and wellness

Date_____

Emotional state

Date_____

Relationships
(friends, family, colleagues, adversaries, general public)

Date_____

Career or work

Date_____

Leisure activities

Date_____

123

Overall level of stress

Date_____

Stop and compare these descriptions with your starting descriptions (beginning on page 2).

Notes